The FODMAP Free

PALEO BREAKTHROUGH™

4 Weeks of Autoimmune Paleo Recipes Without FODMAPS!

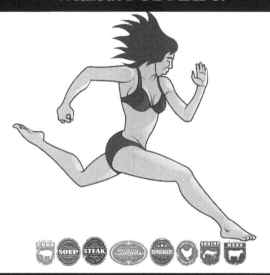

BY ANNE ANGELONE, LICENSED ACUPUNCTURIST

The
FODMAP FREE
Paleo Breakthrough

4 Weeks of Autoimmune Paleo Recipes
Without FODMAPS

by

Anne Angelone

TABLE OF CONTENTS

PREFACE..2

WHAT ARE FODMAPS? 2
WHAT IS FODMAP INTOLERANCE? 2
WHAT CAUSES FODMAP INTOLERANCE? 2
THE AIP AND FODMAP CATEGORIES 3
FODMAPS 5
SIBO 5
FOODS TO INCLUDE IN THE FODMAP FREE AIP MENU PLAN 6
FODMAP FREE PALEO Menu..11

FODMAP FREE PALEO 14

4-Week AIP Menu Plan 14

FODMAP FREE PALEO RECIPES..18

GRILLED TRI-TIP WITH ARUGULA SALAD 18
NEW YORK STEAK AND SPINACH SALAD 19
JUICY PORTERHOUSE STEAK WITH RUSSIAN KALE 19
SKIRT STEAK WITH SAUTEED GREENS..20
BEEF LIVER PATE WITH BACON...20
JUICY GRASS FED BEEF BURGER WITH CRUNCHY GREEN SALAD 21
BALSAMIC PORK TENDERLOIN ON A BED OF RED KALE 21
BALSAMIC MARINATED PORK CHOPS...22
GRILL PAN PORK CHOPS 22
PAN SEARED YELLOWTAIL WITH SAUTEED SPINACH............................23
GINGER STEAMED HALIBUT AND SAUTEED MUSTARD GREENS 23
GRILLED ROSMARY SALMON STEAK WITH STEAMED LACINATO KALE 23
TUNA STEAKS WITH BOK CHOY 24
GRILLED AHI TUNA WITH GINGER AND SAUTÉED RED CHARD.................24
PETRALE SOLE WITH LEMON, OLIVE OIL, THYME AND KALAMATA OLIVES....24
SEARED MACKEREL WITH A SIDE OF MUSTARD GREENS 25
GINGER CILANTRO TUNA STEAK WITH SAUTÉED SPINACH 25
CUCUMBER NORI SALAD 26
BUTTER AND OAK LEAF SALAD 26
DINO KALE AND ORANGE SALAD 27
BACON ARUGULA DAIKON AND CARROT SALAD..................................27
CHICKEN LIVER PATE 28
SLOW COOKED CHICKEN 28
QUICK CHICKEN VEGETABLE SOUP 29
STIR FRIED CHICKEN BREAST WITH YELLOW SUMMER SQUASH...............29
TURMERIC CHICKEN WITH ZUCCHINI AND BASIL 29
BACON WRAPPED CHICKEN THIGHS...30
BLOOD ORANGE CLAY POT CHICKEN 30
OREGANO RUBBED GAME HENS WITH STEAMED RUSSIAN RED KALE 31
GRILLED CHICKEN BREAST WITH KALAMATA OLIVES AND POWER GREENS SALAD.......31
GRILLED CHICKEN WRAPPED IN STEAMED COLLARD GREENS 32
GROUND TURKEY HASH 32
VEGETABLE BROTH 33

CHICKEN STOCK 33
BONE BROTH 34
CARROT GINGER SOUP WITH BACON ON TOP 34
PASTURED TRI-TIP, JUMBO SHRIMP AND COLLARD GREENS 35
JUMBO SHRIMP SAUTEED WITH WATERCRESS 35
SEARED MACKEREL WITH A SIDE OF MUSTARD GREENS 36
STIR FRY SHRIMP, GINGER, CILANTRO, WATER CHESTUNUTS AND BOK CHOY 36
STEAMED ALASKAN KING CRAB WITH SAUTÉED BOK CHOY 37
ROSEMARY AND SEA SALT BAKED LAMB CHOPS ON A BED OF KALE CHIPS 38
SQUASH PASTA WITH TURKEY, BACON, AND GREENS 39
RAW ZUCCHINI NOODLES WITH SEASONED GROUND PORK 39
LEMON COCONUT KEFIR WATER 40
BLUEBERRY COCONUT KEFIR WATER 40
HOMEMADE COCONUT YOGURT 41
VANILLA COCONUT JELLO-GURT 41
CINNAMON COCONUT JELLO-GURT 42
LEMON ORANGE GELATINO 42
BLUEBERRY SPEARMINT GELATINO 42
GREEN SMOOTHIE WITH BLUEBERRY, KALE, GINGER 43
BLUEBERRY, MINT FIZZY 43
GINGER, BLUEBERRY SORBET 43
KIWI, GINGER, MINT SORBET 43
VANILLA, CINNAMON, BANANA SORBET 44
BANANA, STRAWBERRY SORBET 44
GINGER ORANGE, GRAPEFRUIT SORBET 44

QUICK REFERENCE GUIDE 45

SHOPPING LIST 45
WEEK 1 45
GROUND TURKEY HASH 45
GREEN SMOOTHIE WITH BLUEBERRY, KALE, GINGER 45
GINGER STEAMED HALIBUT AND SAUTEED MUSTARD GREENS 45
BLUEBERRY, MINT FIZZY 45
CHICKEN LIVER PATE 46
SEARED MACKEREL WITH A SIDE OF MUSTARD GREENS 46
BONE BROTH 46
SLOW COOKED CHICKEN 46
JUMBO SHRIMP SAUTEED WITH WATERCRESS 47
VEGETABLE BROTH 47
TURMERIC CHICKEN WITH ZUCCHINI AND BASIL 47
BLUEBERRY COCONUT KEFIR WATER 47
GRILLED CHICKEN WRAPPED IN STEAMED COLLARD GREENS 48
BONE BROTH 48
ROSEMARY AND SEA SALT BAKED LAMB CHOPS ON A BED OF KALE CHIPS 48
HOMEMADE COCONUT YOGURT 48
GRILL PAN PORK CHOPS WITH SAUTÉED YELLOW SQUASH AND ARUGULA SALAD 48
GINGER, ORANGE, GRAPEFRUIT SORBET 49
BALSAMIC PORK TENDERLOIN ON A BED OF RED KALE 49
VEGETABLE BROTH 49

HOMEMADE COCONUT YOGURT 49
GINGER CILANTRO TUNA STEAK WITH SAUTÉED SPINACH 49
GREEN SMOOTHIE WITH BLUEBERRY, KALE, GINGER 50
GREEN SMOOTHIE WITH BLUEBERRY, KALE, GINGER 50
BACON ARUGULA DAIKON AND CARROT SALAD......................................50
WEEK 2...50
GRILLED ROSMARY SALMON STEAK WITH STEAMED LACINATO KALE 51
GRILLED CHICKEN BREAST WITH KALAMATA OLIVES AND POWER GREENS SALAD.......51
JUICY GRASS FED BEEF BURGER WITH CRUNCHY GREEN SALAD 51
BONE BROTH 51
BACON WRAPPED CHICKEN THIGHS..52
PAN SEARED YELLOWTAIL WITH SAUTEED SPINACH..................................52
BONE BROTH 52
BALSAMIC MARINATED PORK CHOPS..52
LEMON ORANGE GELATINO 53
RAW ZUCCHINI NOODLES WITH SEASONED GROUND PORK 53
VEGETABLE BROTH 53
TURMERIC CHICKEN WITH ZUCCHINI AND BASIL 53
BACON ARUGULA DAIKON AND CARROT SALAD......................................54
BUTTER AND OAK LEAF SALAD WITH GRILLED ZUCCHINI AND ACV DRESSING.............54
BLUEBERRY SPEARMINT GELATINO 54
GRILLED TRI-TIP WITH ARUGULA SALAD 54
HOMEMADE COCONUT YOGURT 55
BANANA, STRAWBERRY SORBET 55
BONE BROTH 55
STEAMED ALASKAN KING CRAB...55
GROUND TURKEY HASH..55
GRILLED CHICKEN WRAPPED IN STEAMED COLLARD GREENS 56
SQUASH PASTA WITH TURKEY, BACON, AND GREENS 56
HOMEMADE COCONUT YOGURT 56
DINO KALE AND ORANGE SALAD 56
JUICY PORTERHOUSE STEAK WITH RUSSIAN KALE 56
BLUEBERRY, MINT FIZZY 57
WEEK 3...58
HOMEMADE COCONUT YOGURT 58
BUTTER AND OAK LEAF SALAD WITH GRILLED ZUCCHINI AND ACV DRESSING.............58
BACON WRAPPED CHICKEN THIGHS..58
LEMON ORANGE GELATINO 58
GINGER STEAMED HALIBUT AND SAUTEED MUSTARD GREENS 58
BONE BROTH 59
PAN SEARED YELLOWTAIL WITH SAUTEED SPINACH..................................59
TURMERIC CHICKEN WITH ZUCCHINI AND BASIL 59
BONE BROTH 59
BLUEBERRY SPEARMINT GELATINO...60
GINGER CILANTRO TUNA STEAK WITH SAUTÉED SPINACH 60
BLUEBERRY COCONUT KEFIR WATER 60
GRILLED ROSMARY SALMON STEAK WITH STEAMED LACINATO KALE 60
BONE BROTH 60
RAW ZUCCHINI NOODLES WITH SEASONED GROUND PORK 61
HOMEMADE COCONUT YOGURT 61

TUNA STEAKS WITH BOK CHOY 61
LEMON COCONUT KEFIR WATER..61
HOMEMADE COCONUT YOGURT 61
SQUASH PASTA WITH TURKEY, BACON, AND GREENS 61
CHICKEN LIVER PATE..62
BACON WRAPPED CHICKEN THIGHS...62
CUCUMBER NORI SALAD 62
JUICY GRASS FED BEEF BURGER WITH CRUNCHY GREEN SALAD 62
WEEK 4..63
GREEN SMOOTHIE WITH BLUEBERRY, KALE, GINGER 63
CARROT GINGER SOUP WITH BACON ON TOP 63
NEW YORK STEAK AND SPINACH SALAD 63
GROUND TURKEY HASH..64
SKIRT STEAK WITH SAUTEED GREENS...64
BONE BROTH 64
OREGANO RUBBED GAME HENS WITH STEAMED RUSSIAN RED KALE 64
VANILLA COCONUT JELLO-GURT 65
GRILLED CHICKEN BREAST WITH KALAMATA OLIVES AND POWER GREENS SALAD.......65
VEGETABLE BROTH 65
BLOOD ORANGE CLAY POT CHICKEN 65
TUNA STEAKS WITH BOK CHOY 66
HOMEMADE COCONUT YOGURT 66
PETRALE SOLE WITH LEMON, OLIVE OIL, THYME AND KALAMATA OLIVES...................66
CHICKEN LIVER PATE..66
BALSAMIC MARINATED PORK CHOPS WITH MASHED TURNIPS...................................66
CINNAMON COCONUT JELLO-GURT 67
BEEF LIVER PATE WITH BACON 67
GRILLED AHI TUNA WITH GINGERAND SAUTÉED RED CHARD 67
BLUEBERRY SPEARMINT GELATINO..67
PASTURED TRI-TIP, JUMBO SHRIMP AND COLLARD GREENS 68
VEGETABLE BROTH 68
JUMBO SHRIMP SAUTEED WITH WATERCRESS 68
HOMEMADE COCONUT YOGURT 68
STEAMED ALASKAN KING CRAB WITH SAUTÉED BOK CHOY 68
GREEN SMOOTHIE WITH BLUEBERRY, KALE, GINGER 69
BONE BROTH 69
GINGER ORANGE, GRAPEFRUIT SORBET...69
JUICY GRASS FED BEEF BURGER WITH CRUNCHY GREEN SALAD 69
SKIRT STEAK WITH SAUTEED GREENS...69

ABOUT THE AUTHOR **70**

AUTOIMMUNE RESOURCES:...71

COPYRIGHT © BY ANNE ANGELONE 2013

All Rights Reserved

ISBN-13: 978-1492116226

ISBN-10: 149211622X

Images used with permission from 123RF.COM.

Disclaimer: This program manual is not intended to provide medical advice or to take the place of medical advice and treatment from your personal physician. Readers are advised to consult their own doctors or other qualified health professionals regarding the treatment of medical conditions. The author, shall not be held liable or responsible for any misunderstanding or misuse of the information contained in this program manual or for any loss, damage, or injury caused or alleged to be caused directly or indirectly by any treatment, action, or application of any food or food source discussed in this program manual. The U.S Food and Drug Administration have not evaluated contents in this manual. This information is not intended to diagnose, treat, cure, or prevent any disease.

To request permission for reproduction or to inquire about group classes and consulting, please contact:

Anne Angelone, Licensed Acupuncturist

Website: www.paleobreakthrough.com

Preface

WHAT ARE FODMAPS?

FODMAPs is an acronym for fermentable carbohydrates found in common foods. FODMAPs stand for Fermentable Oligosaccharides (fructans and galactans), Disaccharhides (lactose), Monosaccharides (fructose), and Polyols (sugar alcohols).

WHAT IS FODMAP INTOLERANCE?

FODMAP intolerance basically means that fructose and other longer chain carbohydrates are difficult to break down.

When FODMAP foods ferment in the distal small intestine or in the large intestine, they feed bacterial overgrowths, which along with enzyme deficiencies, can cause symptoms like gas, bloating, cramping, diarrhea, constipation, heartburn, excessive burping, depression, fatigue, headache and even brain fog. FODMAP intolerance differs from food sensitivies in that FODMAP foods are just poorly digested versus a being a food that provokes an immune response.

WHAT CAUSES FODMAP INTOLERANCE?

FODMAP intolerance, also referred to as fructose malabsorption, may stem from a deficiency of enzymes that are required to break down longer chain carbohydrates e.g. the oligosaccharide, fructan into shorter chain monosaccharides. Fructose malabsorption may also be due to a lack of a fructose transporter, called GLUT5, which delivers fructose into cells. The sugar alcohols, called Polyols (naturally found in apples, peaches, pears and celery and in "sweeteners" such as sorbitol) can further create digestive distress by blocking this specific fructose transporter GLUT5. In general, those with a GLUT5 deficiency will be more sensitive to fructose and polyols while those with digestive enzyme deficiency are more sensitive to fructans (fructose rich carbs).

Since FODMAP foods generally cause problems in cases of enzyme deficiencies, GLUT5 blocks, dysbiosis and/or small intestine bacterial overgrowth, intolerance to these foods may provide a useful clinical clue about what needs to be corrected.

THE AIP AND FODMAP CATEGORIES

The term autoimmune protocol" or "AIP" has come to refer to a food plan geared toward improving immune function via decreasing triggers, strengthening digestion, and improving overall health. The goal is to increase anti-inflammatory foods to heal the integrity of the gut lining while simultaneously eliminating foods that create low grade immune/inflammatory responses, irritate the gut lining, and feed harmful bacteria (which lead to SIBO and dysbiosis). By eliminating the underlying mechanisms that drive inflammation and autoimmunity, you can modulate and bring balance to your overactive immune system.

The advanced AIP is a great template to begin removing FODMAPs as it already devoid of many disaccharides e.g. lactose (a milk sugar and disaccharide) found in cow, sheep, and goat's milk, as well as many oligosaccharides (e.g fructans found in wheat, inulin, FOS and galactans found in beans and lentils).

The FODMAP Free Paleo menu also excludes:

Excess fructose fruits: e.g. mango, pear, persimmons, pear, watermelon, excess polyol fruits: apple, apricot, avocado, blackberries, cherries, longon, lychee, nectarine, peaches, plums, prunes, excess fructan vegetables: artichokes, asparagus, beet, brussel sprouts, cabbage, chicory, dandelion leaves, fennel, garlic, leek, okra, onions, radicchio and shallots, as well as excess polyol vegetables: avocado, mushrooms, and cauliflower. Fruits that have a 1:1 fructose to glucose ratio are usually well tolerated (e.g. blueberries) but fruits that have more fructose: glucose (e.g apples and pears) tend to be problematic.

If you are having trouble digesting FODMAPs, there are hydrogen breath tests you can order but an elimination diet, such as this FODMAP Free Paleo Menu, may be more reliable to help investigate what you are sensitive to. The very tailored menu plan presented here is based on the advanced autoimmune protocol but goes further by subtracting FODMAPS and even omits starchy foods to starve Small Intestine Bacterial Overgrowth (SIBO).

The FODMAP Free Paleo menu includes 4 weeks of Autoimmune Paleo meals and recipes for those needing to identify FODMAPS that are causing distress while making an effort to starve bacterial overgrowths of any starch or sugars that are found in FODMAP and SIBO caution foods.

Again, it is important to recognize that FODMAP intolerance can indicate either enzyme deficiencies, GLUT5 insufficiency and/or the possibility of having small intestine bacterial overgrowth and/or dysbiosis, which may require further testing and follow up with a qualified health care professional.

This book is dedicated to those who are exploring The Advanced Autoimmune Protocol and have requested a menu plan that excludes FODMAPs and SIBO caution foods. Special thanks to Sarah Ballantyne, Ph.D. aka: The Paleo Mom, for contributing info about FODMAPS and the mechanisms of fructose intolerance and for overall excellence in spreading the word about nutrition for autoimmune conditions. Now, let's get cooking!

NB: In e-book format, all menu options are clickable and hyperlinked to recipe page.

FODMAPS

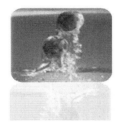

F O D M A P   F O O D S

The FODMAPs in the autoimmune protocol that are eliminated in this 4-week FODMAP Free menu plan are: Apples, artichokes, apricots, asparagus, avocado, beet root, blackberries, broccoli, Brussels sprouts, butternut squash, cabbage, cauliflower, celery, coconut flour, coconut milk, coconut cream, coconut butter, cherries, chicory, dried coconut, dried fruits, fennel bulb, garlic, grapes, honey, longon, lychee, leeks, mushrooms, nectarines, okra, onions, pears, plum, persimmon, peaches, pluots, prunes, pumpkin, radicchio, sauerkraut.

SIBO

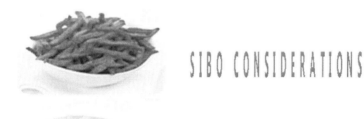

SIBO CONSIDERATIONS

Small Intestine Bacterial Overgrowth (SIBO) is now recognized as a significant yet overlooked cause of IBS. Parsnips, yams, jicama, kohlrabi, okra, sweet potato, taro, plantain, Jerusalem artichoke, lotus root, tapioca, cassava and yucca are generally allowed in the autoimmune protocol but are also avoided in the following menu plan.

FOODS TO INCLUDE IN THE FODMAP FREE AIP MENU PLAN

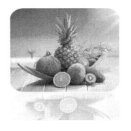

F R U I T S

Bananas, blueberries, cranberry, grapefruit, kiwi, lemons, limes, oranges.

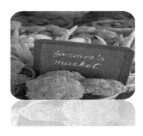

V E G E T A B L E S

Arugula, basil, burdock, bok choy, carrots, chard, collards, cucumber, daikon radish, kale, lettuce, mustard, nettles, purslane, radish, spinach, summer squash, turnips, water chestnuts, watercress, zucchini.

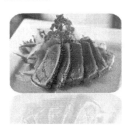

W I L D   F I S H

Salmon, mackerel, herring, halibut, shellfish, oysters, cod, tuna, flounder, sardines, hake, skate, trout, red snapper, etc.

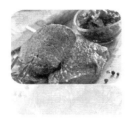

M E A T

Beef, chicken; quail, squab, duck, goose, turkey, Cornish game hen; pasture-raised lamb, pork, buffalo/bison, goat, emu, ostrich, sausage, (without fillers or nightshade spices); liver, kidney, heart, organic sliced meats (gluten, sugar free), uncured nitrate/nitrite-free deli meats and bacon from grass-fed/pastured beef/pork.

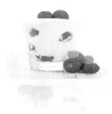

MILK AND YOGURT

Unsweetened coconut yogurt, unsweetened coconut kefir.

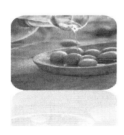

FATS AND OIL

Extra virgin olive oil, red palm oil, tallow from grass-fed beef or lamb, lard from pastured pork.

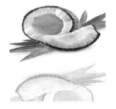

C O C O N U T

Unsweetened coconut yogurt, unsweetened coconut kefir.

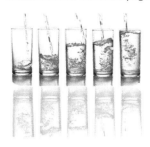

B E V E R A G E S

Filtered or distilled water, herbal tea, mineral water, broths, freshly made veggie juice, green smoothies, kefir water, coconut kefir, kombucha.

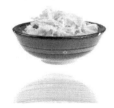

F E R M E N T E D   F O O D S

Coconut yogurt, coconut kefir, kefir water, kombucha.

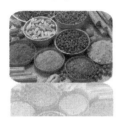

H E R B S   A N D   S P I C E S

Ginger, rosemary, basil, cilantro, dill, lemongrass, peppermint, oregano, parsley, sage, sea salt, thyme, tarragon, turmeric, spearmint, marjoram, mace, chives, chamomile, chervil, cinnamon, bay leaves, cloves, saffron, sea salt.

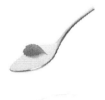

SUGAR SUBSTITUTES

Cinnamon, mint and ginger.

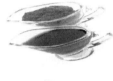

CONDIMENTS

Apple cider vinegar, balsamic vinegar, red boat fish sauce.

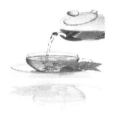

TEA

Herbal teas: peppermint, ginger, lemongrass, spearmint, chamomile, lavender, cinnamon, milk thistle.

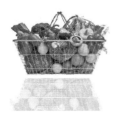 S U P E R   F O O D S

Superfoods to include: bone broth, fermented cod liver oil, gelatin, coconut yogurt, pastured/grass-fed organ meat e.g. liver, wild-caught cold water fish (e.g. salmon, sardines, herring, mackerel), power veggies e.g. kale, chard, spinach, green smoothies.

FODMAP FREE PALEO MENU

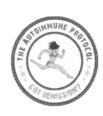
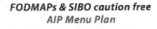

FODMAPs & SIBO caution free
AIP Menu Plan

♯ BEEF

- NEW YORK STEAK AND SPINACH SALAD
- BEEF LIVER PATE WITH BACON
- ARUGULA SALAD WITH GRILLED TRI-TIP
- JUICY GRASS FEDBEEF BURGER WITH POWER GREENS SALAD
- JUICY PORTERHOUSE STEAK WITH RUSSIAN KALE
- PASTURED TRI-TIP, JUMBO SHRIMP AND COLLARD GREENS
- SKIRT STEAK WITH SAUTEED GREENS

♯ POULTRY

- CHICKEN LIVER PATE
- SLOW COOKED CHICKEN
- STIR FRIED CHICKEN WITH YELLOW SUMMER SQUASH AND MINT
- GRILLED CHICKEN WRAPPED IN STEAMED COLLARD GREENS
- BACON WRAPPED CHICKEN THIGHS
- SPAGHETTI SQUASH PASTA WITH TURKEY, BACON AND GREENS
- BLOOD ORANGE CLAY POT CHICKEN
- OREGANO RUBBED CORNISH HENS
- GROUND TURKEY HASH
- GRILLED CHICKEN BREAST WITH KALAMATA OLIVE SPREAD

¤ SEAFOOD

- JUMBO SHRIMP SAUTEED WITH WATERCRESS
- TUNA STEAKS WITH BOK CHOY
- GINGER STEAMED HALIBUT WITH SAUTEED MUSTARD GREENS
- GINGER TUNA STEAK WITH SAUTEED SPINACH
- STEAMED ALASKAN KING CRAB WITH SAUTEED BOK CHOY
- PETRALE SOLE WITH LEMON, CAPERS AND KALAMATA OLIVES
- GRILLED AHI TUNA WITH SEA SALT AND SAUTEED RED CHARD
- GRILLED ROSEMARY SALMON STEAK WITH GINGER AND STEAMED LACINATO KALE
- SEARED MACKEREL WITH A SIDE OF MUSTARD GREEENS
- STIR FRY SHRIMP, GINGER, CILANTRO, WATER CHESTNUTS AND BOK CHOY

¤ LAMB

- ROSEMARY AND SEA SALT BAKED LAMB CHOPS ON A BED OF KALE CHIPS

¤ PORK

- GRILL PAN PORK CHOPS WITH SAUTEED YELLOW SQUASH AND ARUGULA SALAD
- BALSAMIC PORK TENDERLOIN
- RAW ZUCCHINI NOODLES WITH SEASONED GROUND PORK

¤ SALADS

- BUTTER AND OAK LEAF SALAD WITH GRILLED ZUCCHINI AND ACV DRESSING
- BACON ARUGULA DAIKON CARROT SALAD
- CUCUMBER NORI SALAD
- DINO KALE AND ORANGE SALAD

¤ SOUPS

- CARROT GINGER SOUP WITH BACON ON TOP
- CHICKEN VEGETABLE SOUP
- CHICKEN STOCK
- BONE BROTH
- VEGETABLE BROTH

¤ PROBIOTIC FOODS

- HOMEMADE COCONUT YOGURT
- LEMON COCONUT KEFIR WATER
- BLUEBERRY COCONUT KEFIR WATER
- CINNAMON COCONUT JELLO-GURT
- VANILLA COCONUT JELLO-GURT

¤ DESSERTS

- LEMON ORANGE GELATINO
- BLUEBERRY MINT GELATINO
- KIWI, GINGER, MINT SORBET
- VANILLA, CINNAMON, BANANA SORBET
- BANANA, STRAWBERRY SORBET
- GINGER, ORANGE, GRAPEFRUIT SORBET

¤ DRINKS

- GREEN SMOOTHIE WITH BLUEBERRY, KALE, AND GINGER
- BLUEBERRY MINT FIZZY

FODMAP FREE PALEO

4-WEEK AIP MENU PLAN

FODMAP AND SIBO CAUTION FREE

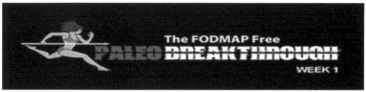

	Breakfast	Snack	Lunch	Snack	Dinner	Beverage
Day 1	Ground Turkey Hash	Green Smoothie	Grilled Tri-Tip with Arugula Salad	Green Salad with cucumber and steamed carrots	Ginger Steamed Halibut with sautéed mustard greens	Blueberry Mint Fizzy
Day 2	Ground beef sautéed in olive oil with salt, oregano, diced carrots and kale	Chicken Liver Pate with carrot sticks	Seared Mackerel with a side of mustard greens	Bone Broth with spinach and basil	Slow cooked Chicken	Water
Day 3	Turkey sausage with steamed bokchoy	Sliced turkey breast with slices of cucumber	Jumbo Shrimp sautéed with watercress	Veggie Broth	Turmeric Chicken with sautéed zucchini	Sparkling Water
Day 4	Ground chicken sautéed with diced carrots, kale, olives	Blueberry Coconut Kefir Water	Grilled Chicken wrapped in steamed collards with crunchy veggies	Bone Broth	Rosemary and Sea Salt Baked Lamb Chops; and arugula salad	Water with 1 Tbsp Apple Cider Vinegar
Day 5	Homemade Coconut Yogurt, with banana and blueberries	Fermented carrots with cucumbers, chicken breast slices	Grill Pan Pork Chops, sautéed yellow squash, mixed green salad	Ginger Grapefruit Sorbet	Balsamic Pork Tenderloin	Mint Tea
Day 6	Pork Sausages sautéed with Swiss chard	Veggie Broth carrots	Crock Pot Chicken	Coconut Yogurt	Tuna Steak spinach and romaine salad	Green Smoothie
Day 7	Roast beef slices, Green Smoothie	Bacon spinach salad with grated carrot, balsamic, olive oil, sea salt	Bacon, Arugula, Daikon and Carrot Salad	Chicken breast slices	Grilled Rosemary Salmon Steak with steamed Lacinato kale	Kombucha

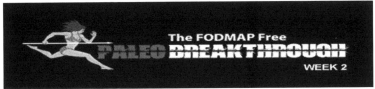

	Breakfast	Snack	Lunch	Snack	Dinner	Beverage
Day 1	Grilled Rosemary Salmon Steak with steamed Lacinato kale	Orange slices, 2 oz. grilled chicken breast	Juicy Grilled Grass Fed Beef	Bone Broth	Bacon Wrapped Chicken Thighs and sautéed mustard greens	Kombucha
Day 2	Chicken sausage sautéed with water chestnuts and Swiss chard	Cucumber with sea salt, turkey breast	Pan Seared Yellowtail	Bone Broth	Balsamic Marinated Pork Chop with mashed turnips and sautéed greens	Water with Lemon
Day 3	Chicken breast sautéed with bokchoy	Lemon Orange Gelatino	Raw zucchini noodles with seasoned ground pork	Veggie Broth	Turmeric Chicken with zucchini and butter leaf salad	Ginger Tea
Day 4	Turkey burger with sautéed Rainbow chard	Bacon, Arugula, Daikon and Carrot Salad	Butter and Oak Leaf Salad with grilled zucchini and ACV Dressing	Blueberry Mint Gelatino	Arugula Salad with Grilled Tri-Tip	Water with Apple Cider Vinegar
Day 5	Homemade Coconut Yogurt Blueberries	Banana Strawberry Sorbet	Fresh turkey breast slices; Carrot sticks	Bone Broth	Alaskan King Crab with sautéed BokChoy	Lavender, Mint Tea
Day 6	Ground Turkey Hash	Freshly made carrot, ginger juice	Grilled Chicken Wrapped in steamed collard with crunchy veggies	Green Salad with cucumber and steamed carrots	Spaghetti Squash & Spinach with ground turkey and bacon	Water
Day 7	Chicken Soup with cilantro on top	Coconut Kefir smoothie with bananas	Dino Kale with orange salad	A few slices of Turkey; cucumbers	Juicy Porterhouse Steak with Russian Red Kale	Blueberry mint fizzy

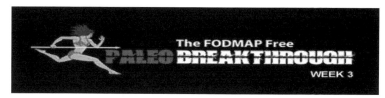

	Breakfast	Snack	Lunch	Snack	Dinner	Beverage
Day 1	Homemade Coconut Yogurt with cinnamon, banana	Freshly made carrot, ginger juice	Butter and Oak Leaf Salad with grilled zucchini and ACV Dressing	Sardines in endive	Bacon Wrapped Chicken Thighs with steamed Butternut squash and sautéed mustard greens	Nettle
Day 2	Ground chicken sautéed with diced carrots, Kale, olives	Lemon Orange Gelatino	Ginger Steamed Halibut with sautéed mustard greens	Bone Broth	Pan Seared Yellowtail with sautéed spinach	Water
Day 3	Turmeric Chicken with zucchini and butter leaf salad	Bone Broth	Chicken Vegetable Soup	Blueberry Mint Gelatino	Ginger Tuna with sautéed spinach	Kombucha
Day 4	2 Turkey patties with sautéed Rainbow chard	Blueberry Coconut Kefir water	Grilled Rosemary Salmon Steak with steamed Lacinato kale	Bone Broth	Raw Zucchini Noodles with seasoned ground pork	Water with 1 Tbsp Apple Cider Vinegar
Day 5	Homemade Coconut Yogurt with cinnamon, maple syrup	Bright green olives	Fresh turkey breast slices; Carrot sticks	Turkey Sausage	Tuna Steaks with Bok Choy	Mint Tea
Day 6	Chicken sausages with steamed carrots and kale	Lemon Kefir water	Carrot Ginger Soup with Bacon on Top	Homemade coconut yogurt, banana	Squash Pasta with Turkey, Bacon and Greens	Lemon Water
Day 7	Chicken liver pâté. Steamed leafy greens	Fermented carrots, and chicken breast	Bacon Wrapped Chicken Thighs and sautéed mustard greens	Cucumber Nori Salad	Juicy Grilled Grass Fed Beef	Kombucha

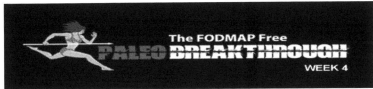

	Breakfast	Snack	Lunch	Snack	Dinner	Beverage
Day 1	Chicken Breast sautéed with Zucchini and Basil	Green Smoothie kale, blueberries and ginger	Carrot Ginger Soup with chopped bacon on top	Green Smoothie of kale, blueberries and ginger	New York Steak with sautéed collard greens	Kombucha
Day 2	Ground Turkey Hash	Turkey breast, raw carrots	Skirt Steak with sautéed greens	Bone broth	Oregano Rubbed Game Hens with steamed Russian red kale and oak leaf salad	Water
Day 3	Vanilla Coconut Jellogurt with blueberries	Chicken Broth with fresh dill	Grilled Chicken with kalamata olives and power greens salad	Vegetable Broth	Blood Orange Clay Pot Chicken with turnips, carrots and leeks	Kombucha
Day 4	Tuna Steak Sautéed spinach	Coconut yogurt smoothie with blueberries	Petrale Sole sautéed with lemon, olive oil and kalamata olives	Chicken Liver Pate on endive with capers on top	Balsamic Marinated Pork Chops with mashed turnips and sautéed greens	Water with 1 TBSP Apple Cider Vinegar
Day 5	Cinnamon Coconut Yogurt, with banana	Beef Liver Pate with Bacon in romaine hearts	Grilled Ahi Tuna with ginger and red chard	Blueberry Mint Gelatino	Pastured Tri-Tip, Jumbo Shrimp and collard greens	Chamomile Tea
Day 6	Chicken sausages served with steamed chard, kale, mustard drizzled with olive oil, salt to taste	Veggie broth, carrots	Jumbo Shrimp sautéed with watercress	Homemade Coconut Yogurt with blueberries	Alaskan King Crab with sautéed bok choy	Green Smoothie
Day 7	Roast beef slices, sautéed spinach, Bone Broth	Ginger Orange Grapefruit Sorbet	Grass Fed Bacon Burgers with romaine salad	A couple slices of roast beef with raw carrots	Skirt Steak with sautéed greens	Kombucha

Recipes

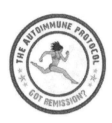

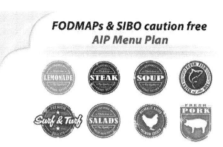

**FODMAPs & SIBO caution free
AIP Menu Plan**

GRILLED TRI-TIP WITH ARUGULA SALAD

- 4 cups fresh arugula
- 1 carrot peeled and grated
- 2 Tbsp olive oil
- 2 Tbsp balsamic vinegar
- Sea salt to taste
- ½ pound Tri-tip steak

Preparation

1. Mix arugula with grated carrots in a large bowl.
2. Stir in the olive oil, vinegar, salt, and Adjust seasonings.
3. Sprinkle salt on tri-tip steak and cook on grill pan for 7-10 minutes on each side. Slice thinly and serve on top of salad

Servings: 1-2

NEW YORK STEAK AND SPINACH SALAD

- 1 pound New York Steak
- 1 head of washed spinach
- 1 carrot peeled and grated
- ½ peeled and sliced cucumber
- 2 Tbsp olive oil
- 2 Tbsp balsamic vinegar
- Sea salt to taste
- Olive oil spray

Preparation

1. Mix spinach with grated carrots in a large bowl.
2. Stir in olive oil, vinegar, and salt.
3. Sprinkle sea salt and spray olive oil on New York Steak, cook on grill pan for 7 minutes per side. Slice and serve over salad.

Servings: 2

JUICY PORTERHOUSE STEAK WITH RUSSIAN KALE

- One 1 pound porterhouse steak
- 4 cups Russian red kale
- 4 Tbsp olive oil
- Olive oil spray
- Sea salt to taste

Preparation

1. Sautee kale in olive oil with sea salt to taste.
2. Sprinkle sea salt on meat and spray with olive oil.
3. Cook on grill pan for 10 minutes per side or to desired doneness.

Servings: 2

SKIRT STEAK WITH SAUTEED GREENS

- 1 bunch of mustard greens, chopped
- 1 pound of skirt steak
- 4 Tbsp olive oil, divided
- Sea salt to taste

Preparation

1. Lightly salt skirt steak and grill for 10 minutes on each side.
2. Sautee mustard greens in 4 Tbsp olive oil

Servings: 1-2

BEEF LIVER PATE WITH BACON

- 3/4 pound beef liver
- 1/3 cup olive oil, more to taste
- 2 Tbsp capers
- 3 tsp fresh thyme
- 2 tsp fresh rosemary
- 3 strips of bacon
- 1 Tbsp lemon juice
- Sea salt to taste

Preparation

1. Cook and chop bacon, set aside
2. Sautee beef liver in olive oil
3. Add herbs, capers, lemon juice and simmer until liquid is almost gone.
4. Add salt to taste, blend with bacon in Cuisinart, refrigerate.

Servings 4-5

JUICY GRASS FED BEEF BURGER WITH CRUNCHY GREEN SALAD

- ½ pound ground beef
- Red leaf lettuce and romaine hearts
- 1 peeled and grated carrot
- 2 Tbsp olive oil
- 2 Tbsp balsamic vinegar
- Sea salt to taste

Preparation

1. Grill 2 burgers for 7 minutes on each side.
2. Toss red leaf lettuce, romaine hearts carrots in a large bowl.
3. Stir in the olive oil, vinegar, salt.
4. Optional: Top with bacon

BALSAMIC PORK TENDERLOIN ON A BED OF RED KALE

- 1 teaspoon salt
- 1/4 cup balsamic vinegar
- 1/2 cup olive oil
- 1 one pound pork tenderloin
- 6 leaves of Russian red kale

Preparation

1. Marinate pork for at least one hour and up to 24 hours in above ingredients.
2. Preheat oven to 450 F.
3. Spray olive oil in a baking dish.
4. Massage kale leaves with olive oil and a sprinkle of salt.
5. Pan sear the tenderloin in a skillet for about 3 minutes, browning on all sides, then place on top of kale.
6. Bake in oven at for 15-25 minutes or to desired doneness.
7. Be sure to eat the kale chips!

BALSAMIC MARINATED PORK CHOPS WITH MASHED TURNIPS AND SAUTÉED COLLARDS

- 1 teaspoon sea salt
- 1/4 cup balsamic vinegar
- 6 Tbsp olive oil divided
- 2 bone in one pork chops
- 1 bunch of collard greens
- 4 turnip, boiled until soft
- Sea salt to taste

Preparation

1. Marinate chops for at least one and up to 24 hours in balsamic vinegar and 2 Tbsp Olive oil.
2. Grill 7 minutes per side, checking for doneness
3. While turnips are boiling, sauté the collard greens in olive oil.
4. Mash turnip, add a dash of olive oil and salt to taste

GRILL PAN PORK CHOPS

With sautéed yellow squash and arugula salad

- 2 Pork Chops
- 5 small yellow squash sliced
- ¼ bunch of fresh flat leaf parsley
- 5 Tbsp olive oil divided
- 2 Tbsp balsamic vinegar
- 4 cups arugula
- Sea salt to taste

Preparation

1. Mix thyme with olive oil and salt to rub chops.
2. Grill on med-high heat for 5-7 minutes per side.
3. Sautee yellow squash in olive oil with parsley.
4. Mix arugula with 2 Tbsp olive oil and 2 Tbsp balsamic vinegar.

Servings: 2

PAN SEARED YELLOWTAIL WITH SAUTEED SPINACH

- 1 pound yellow tail
- 2 Tbsp olive or red palm oil
- 1 bunch of spinach
- 1 Tbsp minced ginger
- Sea salt to taste

Preparation

1. Marinate yellowtail in ginger and olive oil for 1 hour.
2. Sautee spinach in olive oil with salt to taste.
3. Spray and preheat skillet on med-high for 3 minutes.
4. Add yellow tail and cook for one minute per ½ inch of thickness,

GINGER STEAMED HALIBUT AND SAUTEED MUSTARD GREENS

- 1 pound halibut
- 1 inch of sliced ginger
- ¼ bunch cilantro
- Lemon slices
- 2 Tbsp olive or red palm oil
- Sea salt to taste
- One bunch of mustard greens

Preparation

1. Cover halibut with olive oil, cilantro, lemon and ginger.
2. Steam the fish for 15 minutes.
3. Sauté mustard greens in olive oil, add salt to taste.

Servings: 2

GRILLED ROSMARY SALMON STEAK WITH STEAMED LACINATO KALE

- 1 bunch Lacinato aka Dino kale
- 1 pound salmon
- 2 sprigs rosemary
- 2 Tbsp olive or red palm oil
- Olive oil spray
- Sea salt to taste

Preparation

1. Coat the salmon with olive oil spray, a light dusting of salt and crushed rosemary. Grill for 8 minutes on each side.
2. Steam kale and serve.

Servings: 2

TUNA STEAKS WITH BOK CHOY

- 1 bunch bok choy
- 1 pound tuna steaks
- 2 Tbsp olive or red palm oil
- Sea salt to taste

Preparation

1. Wash, cut and sauté bok choy in olive oil, sea salt to taste.
2. Coat tuna steaks with olive spray and sea salt
3. Grill for 5 minutes on each side

Servings: 1-2

GRILLED AHI TUNA WITH GINGER AND SAUTÉED RED CHARD

- 1 one pound Ahi tuna steak
- 1 Tbsp minced ginger
- 5+ Tbsp olive or red palm oil, divided
- 1 bunch red chard, chopped

Preparation

1. Marinate Ahi in 2 Tbsp olive oil and ginger for 1 hour or longer.
2. Sautee red chard in 3+ Tbsp olive oil
3. Grill tuna for 6 minutes each side or to desired doneness.

PETRALE SOLE WITH LEMON, OLIVE OIL, THYME AND KALAMATA OLIVES

- 1 1/2 pounds fresh Petrale sole fillets
- 20 kalamata olive, pitted, chopped
- 2 Tbsp olive oil
- Fresh thyme leaves
- Lemon wedges

Preparation

1. Pat the sole fillets dry with paper towels. Lightly salt the fillets on both sides.
2. Heat oil on medium-high heat. Brown the fillets gently on both sides for no more than a few minutes on each side.
3. Add kalamata olives to the pan and sauté with herbs, and a squeeze of lemon juice into the sauce. Drizzle sauce over fish.

Enjoy!

SEARED MACKEREL WITH A SIDE OF MUSTARD GREENS

- 1 pound mackerel
- 2 Tbsp ginger, chopped
- 4 cups mustard greens
- 4Tbsp olive or red palm oil divided
- Olive oil spray
- 2 Tbsp fresh cilantro (chopped)
- Pinch of sea salt

Preparation

1. Marinate mackerel in 2Tbsp oil and ginger
2. Sautee mustard in 2 Tbsp oil, sea salt to taste.
3. Spray olive oil on grill pan
4. Grill mackerel for 5 minutes on each side.

Servings: 1-2

GINGER CILANTRO TUNA STEAK WITH SAUTÉED SPINACH

- Two 4 oz. tuna steaks (1 inch thick)
- 2 tbsp ginger
- 4 cups spinach
- 2 Tbsp olive oil

- Olive oil spray
- 2 Tbsp fresh cilantro (chopped)
- Pinch of sea salt

Preparation

1. Coat tuna steaks with olive oil spray and sea salt
2. Grill for 5 minutes on each side
3. Sautee spinach in olive oil, sea salt to taste

Servings: 1-2

CUCUMBER NORI SALAD

- 2 Nori sheets
- 1 cucumber, peeled, seeded and sliced thin
- 2 Tbsp apple cider vinegar
- 1 tsp ginger root, chopped
- Juice of ½ a lime
- I carrot sliced thin
- 1 Tbsp olive oil
- Sea salt to taste

Preparation

1. Prepare carrot, ginger and cucumber.
2. Cut Nori into thin strips and let sit in a bowl of warm water.
3. Combine olive oil, sea salt and apple cider vinegar.
4. Pour over cut veggies, remove Nori from water and add to salad.

Servings: 1-2

BUTTER AND OAK LEAF SALAD WITH GRILLED ZUCCHINI AND ACV DRESSING

- 1 head of butter leaf lettuce
- 1 head of oak leaf lettuce
- 2 Tbsp apple cider vinegar
- 3 Tbsp olive oil, divided
- Sea salt to taste
- 2 medium zucchinis sliced

Preparation

1. Mix oak leaf and butter leaf lettuce with grated daikon and carrots.
2. Stir in the olive oil, vinegar, salt and adjust seasonings.
3. Sprinkle salt and oil on zucchinis and cook on grill pan until tender.
4. Add to salad, toss and serve.

Servings: 1-2

DINO KALE AND ORANGE SALAD

- 1/2 head of kale
- 1 orange, wedges cut in thirds
- 2 Tbsp olive oil
- 1 tsp sea salt
- 1 Tbsp apple cider vinegar

BACON ARUGULA DAIKON AND CARROT SALAD

- 2 strips of bacon, cooked and chopped
- 1 head of arugula
- 1 small daikon radish, grated
- 1 carrot, grated
- 2 Tbsp olive oil
- 1 tsp sea salt
- 1 Tbsp apple cider vinegar

Preparation

1. Mix arugula with grated daikon, carrots in a large bowl.
2. Stir in the olive oil, vinegar, salt and adjust seasonings.

Servings: 1-2

CHICKEN LIVER PATE

- 1 pound chicken livers
- 1/2 cup olive oil
- 2 tbsp capers
- 3 tsp fresh thyme
- 2 tsp fresh rosemary
- ¼ cup chicken broth or water
- Sea salt to taste

Preparation

1. Sauté chicken livers in olive oil until brown.
2. Add broth, herbs, capers and simmer until liquid is mostly gone.
3. Add salt to taste, blend in Cuisinart, refrigerate.

SLOW COOKED CHICKEN

- 3 Lbs boneless, skinless chicken thighs
- 3 carrots, chopped
- Sea salt to taste
- 2 medium zucchinis chopped
- 1/4 cup olive oil
- 1 TB dried thyme
- 1 TB sage
- 1 1/2 cups chicken broth

Preparation

1. Add everything to your slow cooker or crock-pot and let cook on medium-high for 4 hours.

QUICK CHICKEN VEGETABLE SOUP

- 1 container chicken broth
- 1 grilled and sliced chicken breast
- ½ head of Dino kale
- 2 Tbsp olive oil
- 1 sliced carrot
- ¼ bunch cilantro
- Sea salt to taste

Preparation

1. Sautee kale and carrot in olive oil.
2. Stir in the chicken broth; add salt, sliced chicken and cilantro.

Servings: 1-2

STIR FRIED CHICKEN BREAST WITH YELLOW SUMMER SQUASH AND MINT IN BUTTER LEAF LETTUCE WRAP

- 2 chicken breasts
- 3 medium zucchinis, sliced thinly
- 1/2 bunch of mint
- 4 Tbsp olive oil
- Olive oil spray
- Sea salt to taste
- 1 head of butter leaf lettuce

Preparation

1. Cut chicken into cubes and sauté in olive oil, pinch of salt.
2. After 5 minutes add zucchini in olive oil and sauté for 7 minutes
3. Fill butter leaf lettuce with chicken sauté and fresh mint, serve.

Servings: 2-3

TURMERIC CHICKEN WITH ZUCCHINI AND BASIL

- 2 grilled chicken breasts
- 3 medium zucchinis, sliced thinly
- ½ bunch of basil leaves
- 2 Tbsp olive oil
- 2 tsp turmeric
- Olive oil spray
- Sea salt to taste

Preparation

1. Coat chicken breasts with olive oil spray and salt and turmeric. Grill for 8-10 minutes on each side.
2. Sautee zucchini in olive oil for 10 minutes and add basil in last 2 minutes.
3. Slice chicken and serve with sautéed zucchini.

Servings: 2

BACON WRAPPED CHICKEN THIGHS

- 4 pieces of boneless, skinless chicken thighs
- 4 pieces of bacon
- 3 Tbsp olive oil
- 1 tsp sea salt

Preparation

1. Preheat the oven to 375 F.
2. Coat chicken with olive oil and salt, fold in half then wrap
3. One piece of bacon around each chicken thigh.
4. Bake for 30 minutes. Broil the chicken for another 5-10 minutes or until the bacon is crispy and the chicken is fully cooked.

Servings: 2

BLOOD ORANGE CLAY POT CHICKEN

- One 3 pound chicken
- Juice of 1 lemon
- 1 blood orange, cut in half
- 3 Tbsp olive oil
- 5 sprigs of thyme, leaves pulled and chopped
- 5 sprigs of thyme for inside cavity
- 1 turnip cubed
- 2 carrots, peeled and cut in quarters
- Sea salt to taste

Preparation

1. Soak clay pot roaster in cold water for 15 minutes.
2. Mix thyme, lemon juice and olive oil.
3. Rinse chicken, pat dry then rub with salt, thyme and olive oil mix.
4. Cut turnips and carrots, coat with olive oil, sea salt to taste.

5. Place chicken on top of veggies in clay pot.
6. Squeeze the juice of one blood orange on top of chicken and veggies then place in cavity with lemon and thyme.
7. Cover clay pot and place in cold oven
8. Raise temp to 400F and bake for 75 minutes, making sure chicken is cooked.

Servings: 4

OREGANO RUBBED GAME HENS WITH STEAMED RUSSIAN RED KALE AND OAK LEAF SALAD

- 2 Cornish Hens (approx 1 lb. each)
- 1 Tbsp olive oil
- Sea salt
- 3/4 bunch of fresh oregano, chopped
- ¼ bunch oregano set aside for cavity
- 1 bunch Russian red kale
- ½ pound of Oak Leak salad
- 4 sprigs of rosemary

Preparation

1. Preheat oven to 450F
2. Rinse hen, pat dry then rub with oil, salt, oregano blend.
3. Place 1 lemon wedge and 3 sprigs of oregano in cavity of each hen.
4. Put in roasting pan and cook at 450F for 25 minutes
5. Reduce heat to 350.
6. Mix chicken broth, and remaining 2 tablespoons of oil; pour over hens.
7. Continue roasting about 25 minutes longer, or until hens are golden brown.
8. Cut hens lengthwise and serve.

GRILLED CHICKEN BREAST WITH KALAMATA OLIVES AND POWER GREENS SALAD

- 2 chicken breasts
- 20 kalamata olives, pitted and chopped
- 3 Tbsp olive oil
- Fresh thyme leaves for 3 sprigs

- Olive oil spray
- 2 Tbsp apple cider vinegar
- ¼ bunch ea. of kale, chard, cilantro

Preparation

1. Coat the chicken with olive oil spray, salt and thyme.
2. Heat oil on medium-high heat.
3. Add kalamata olives to the pan and sauté. Toss greens with olive oil, apple cider vinegar and salt to taste.

GRILLED CHICKEN WRAPPED IN STEAMED COLLARD GREENS WITH CRUNCHY VEGGIES

- 2 chicken breasts
- 1 Tbsp minced ginger
- 3 large carrots, peeled and diced
- Sea salt
- 2 Tbsp olive oil
- ½ daikon radish, peeled and diced
- 1 bunch of collard greens

Preparation

1. Marinate chicken breast in olive oil and ginger for 1 hour or longer.
2. Cut veggies, steam collard greens
3. Grill chicken breasts for 12 minutes each side making sure thoroughly cooked.

GROUND TURKEY HASH

- ½ pound ground turkey
- 1 Tbsp minced ginger
- 2 large carrots, peeled and diced
- Sea salt
- 2 Tbsp olive oil
- 7 water chestnuts

Preparation

1. Sautee ginger for 1-2 minutes in olive oil.
2. Add turkey with carrot and water chestnuts.
3. Add salt to taste, serve.

VEGETABLE BROTH

- 3 quarts of water
- 2 sliced carrots
- 1 cup of cubed daikon
- 1 cup of turnips and rutabaga cut into large cubes
- 2 cups of chopped greens: kale, parsley, collard greens, chard, cilantro
- 4 ½ inch slices of ginger

Preparation

1. Add all the ingredients at once and place on low boil for 60 minutes.
2. Cool and strain veggies out-discard them.
3. Store in fridge. Heat and drink 3-4 cups/day.

Servings: 8 cups

CHICKEN STOCK

- 2 ½ pounds bony chicken pieces
- 2 peeled and chopped carrots
- 1 peeled and chopped daikon
- 2 bay leaves
- 2 quarts of water
- Sea salt to taste
- ¼ bunch fresh thyme leaves

Preparation

1. Add veggies, chicken and herbs to 2 quarts of water in a large pot.
2. Cook for 2 hours.
3. When cool, pour through a strainer to enjoy clear broth

BONE BROTH

- 4 quarts water
- 2 lbs chicken or beef bones
- 2 bay leaves
- 2 tablespoon apple cider vinegar
- 1 teaspoon sea salt

Preparation

1. Place all ingredients in pot and bring the stock to a boil, then reduce the heat to low and allow the stock to cook for 8 -24 hours, adding water as necessary.
2. Allow the stock to cool then strain to discard bones etc.
3. Store your stock in the fridge and use within a few days.

Servings: 1-2

CARROT GINGER SOUP WITH BACON ON TOP

- 3 Tbsp olive oil
- 7 large carrots, peeled and sliced thin
- Sea salt
- 1 teaspoon minced ginger
- 2 cups or vegetable or chicken stock
- 2 cups water
- 3 large strips of zest from an orange
- Chopped parsley, dill and bacon for garnish

Servings: 1-2

Preparation

1. Sautee carrots in olive oil.
2. Add stock, water, ginger and orange zest.
3. Bring to a simmer, cover and cook for 20 minutes.
4. Remove orange zest strips
5. Pour soup in a blender and puree until smooth.
6. Add salt to taste and garnish with bacon, parsley, and dill.

PASTURED TRI-TIP, JUMBO SHRIMP AND COLLARD GREENS

- 1 pound tri-tip steak
- ½ pound pre-cooked shrimp
- 1 bunch of collard greens, rolled then cut thin
- 5 Tbsp olive oil
- Sea salt to taste

Preparation

1. Lightly salt tri-tip and grill for 7 minutes on each side.
2. Sautee collard greens in olive oil for a few minutes, then add shrimp for 5 minutes.
3. Sprinkle salt on tri-tip and cook on grill pan. Serve!
4. Eat like a Queen

Servings: 1-2

JUMBO SHRIMP SAUTEED WITH WATERCRESS

- 1/2 cup chicken stock or broth
- 1/4 cup Red Boat fish sauce
- 5 tablespoons olive oil
- 1 1/4 pounds shelled and deveined jumbo shrimp
- 3 tablespoons minced fresh ginger
- One 6-ounce bunch watercress
- 1 tablespoon fresh lime juice

Preparation

1. In a small bowl, whisk together the stock, fish sauce.
2. In a wok or large skillet, heat 2 tablespoons of olive oil. Add shrimp and cook over high heat, turning once, about 1 minute per side. Transfer to a plate.
3. Add the remaining 3 tablespoons of oil to the skillet. Add ginger and stir-fry over high heat until fragrant, about 1 minute.
4. Stir the stock mixture, add it to the skillet and bring to a boil. Stir in the watercress, then the shrimp and lime juice. Transfer the stir-fry to bowls.

SEARED MACKEREL WITH A SIDE OF MUSTARD GREENS

- 1 pound mackerel
- 2 Tbsp ginger
- 4 cups mustard greens
- 4 Tbsp olive or red palm oil (divided)
- Olive oil spray
- 2 Tbsp fresh cilantro (chopped)
- Pinch of sea salt

Preparation

1. Marinate mackerel in 2 Tbsp oil., ginger.
2. Grill for 5 minutes on each side.
3. Sautee mustard greens2 Tbsp oil.
4. Sea salt to taste.

Servings: 1-2

STIR FRY SHRIMP, GINGER, CILANTRO, WATER CHESTUNUTS AND BOK CHOY

- 1 1/4 pounds shelled and deveined medium shrimp
- 1/2 cup chicken stock or broth
- 10 water chestnuts, sliced
- 6 tablespoons red palm oil
- 3 tablespoons minced fresh ginger
- One head of bok choy
- 1 tablespoon fresh lime juice
- ½ bunch of chopped cilantro

Preparation

1. In a large skillet, heat 3 tablespoons of red palm oil.
2. Add shrimp and cook over high heat, about 1 minute per side. Transfer to a plate.
3. Add the remaining 3 tablespoons of oil to the skillet. Add ginger and cilantro then stir-fry over high heat until fragrant, about 1 minute.
4. Stir the stock mixture, add it to the skillet and bring to a boil. Stir in the bok choy, water chestnuts then shrimp and lime juice. Transfer the stir-fry to bowls.

STEAMED ALASKAN KING CRAB WITH SAUTÉED BOK CHOY

- Alaskan king crab claws
- One bunch of bok choy
- ½ bunch of cilantro chopped
- 6 Tbsp red palm oil, divided
- Sea salt to taste

Preparation

1. Chop cilantro and mix or blend with 3 Tbsp red palm oil.
2. Bring a large pot of water to a boil. Place thawed or fresh crab in a steamer for 10 minutes. Then crack them open and drizzle with red palm oil, cilantro blend.
3. Sautee bok choy in 3 Tbsp. add salt to taste and serve with King Crab.

Servings: 1-2

ROSEMARY AND SEA SALT BAKED LAMB CHOPS ON A BED OF KALE CHIPS WITH ARUGULA AND ENDIVE SALAD

- 1 pound lamb chops
- 2 Tbsp minced fresh rosemary
- 2 teaspoons sea salt
- 4 Tbsp olive oil, divided
- 5 pieces of kale
- Olive oil spray
- 1 head of arugula
- 6 heads of endive, chopped
- 1 cucumber, sliced
- 1 Tbsp. balsamic vinegar

Preparation

1. Preheat oven to 375F.
2. Rub chops with olive oil, rosemary and sea salt.
3. Spray olive oil in a baking dish.
4. Coat 5 large kale leaves with olive oil.
5. Place lamb chops on top of kale.
6. Bake in oven @ 375F for 20 minutes, turn chops over, and cook for 20 more minutes, or to desired doneness.
7. Toss arugula, endive and cucumber with olive oil and sea salt to taste.
8. Be sure to eat the kale chips!

Servings: 2-3

SQUASH PASTA WITH TURKEY, BACON, AND GREENS

- One medium spaghetti squash
- 4 cups packed spinach
- 2 strips of bacon
- 5 Tbsp olive oil, divided
- ½ pound ground turkey meat
- 1 tsp dried oregano
- 1 tsp dried basil
- Sea salt to taste

Preparation

1. Cook and chop bacon, set aside.
2. Sauté spinach in 2 Tbsp olive oil, set aside.
3. Cut the spaghetti squash in half from top to bottom.
4. Remove the seeds from the middle of the squash.
5. Place squash in a steamer for 20 minutes.
6. Add 3 Tbsp. olive oil and oregano in medium sized skillet on med-high.
7. Place the ½ pound of ground turkey in the skillet, breaking pieces apart. Make sure turkey is thoroughly cooked then add in bacon.
8. Once squash is tender, allow it to cool enough to remove insides of the squash. After all of the squash has been removed, place it in the skillet and mix together with turkey, bacon and greens. Mangia!

Servings: 2

RAW ZUCCHINI NOODLES WITH SEASONED GROUND PORK

- 2 large zucchinis, julienned
- ½ pound ground pork
- ¼ bunch chopped fresh basil
- ¼ bunch chopped fresh oregano
- Sea salt to taste
- 3 Tbsp olive oil

Preparation

1. Sautee basil, oregano and pork in olive oil until fully cooked, add salt to taste.
2. Pour on top of zucchini pasta; add more fresh basil, Enjoy!

Servings: 1-2

LEMON COCONUT KEFIR WATER

- 1 quart coconut water
- ½ cup whole lemon
- 3 Tbsp dairy free water kefir grains

Preparation

1. Purchase non-dairy water kefir grains.
2. Place water kefir grains in coconut water.
3. Cover and set aside for 24 hours.
4. Remove the kefir grains.
5. Puree lemon with coconut kefir water in a blender.

BLUEBERRY COCONUT KEFIR WATER

- 1 quart coconut water
- 1 cup blueberries
- 3 Tbsp dairy free water kefir grains

Preparation

1. Purchase non-dairy water kefir grains.
2. Place water kefir grains in coconut water.
3. Cover and set aside for 24 hours.
4. Remove the kefir grains.
5. Puree blueberries with coconut kefir water in a blender.

HOMEMADE COCONUT YOGURT

- 1-quart coconut milk
- ¼ tsp probiotic yogurt starter
- Yogurt maker

Preparation

1. Heat a quart of unsweetened coconut milk to 105F - 110F.
2. Add ¼ teaspoon of yogurt starter and pulse 2x with the blender. You can add more than 1/4 teaspoon per quart if a very firm yogurt is desired.
3. Plug in your yogurt maker and pour the mixture into your yogurt maker container or containers and ferment for 12 hours.
4. Place in refrigerator for 4 hours.

VANILLA COCONUT JELLO-GURT

- 1-quart coconut milk
- ¼ tsp probiotic yogurt starter
- 1 packet of unflavored gelatin
- Yogurt maker
- ¼ tsp vanilla extract

Preparation

1. Heat a quart of unsweetened coconut milk to 105F - 110F.
2. Add ¼ teaspoon of yogurt starter and 1 packet of unflavored gelatin.
3. Pulse 2x with the blender. Plug in your yogurt maker and pour the mixture into your yogurt maker containers and ferment for 12 hours.
4. Place in refrigerator for 4 hours.

CINNAMON COCONUT JELLO-GURT

- 1-quart coconut milk
- ¼ tsp probiotic yogurt starter
- 1 packet of unflavored gelatin
- Yogurt maker
- 1/2 tsp cinnamon

Preparation

1. Heat a quart of unsweetened coconut milk to 105F - 110F.
2. Add ¼ teaspoon of yogurt starter and 1 packet of unflavored gelatin.
3. Pulse 2x with the blender. Plug in your yogurt maker and pour the mixture into your yogurt maker containers and ferment for 12 hours.
4. Place in refrigerator for 4 hours.

LEMON ORANGE GELATINO

- Juice from 1 orange
- 1 tsp lemon zest
- 1 tsp grated orange zest
- 1 cup boiling water
- 4 Tbsp unflavored gelatin

Preparation

1. Mix orange juice, lemon and orange zest, set aside.
2. Add 1 cup boiling water to 4 tablespoons of gelatin in a bowl.
3. Strain lemon and orange zest from juice and add to gelatin.
4. Pour into a glass dish or molds and refrigerate for 60 minutes.

BLUEBERRY SPEARMINT GELATINO

- 1 cup blueberries
- 1/2 cup lemon juice
- ¼ bunch spearmint leaves, chopped
- 4 Tbsp unflavored gelatin

Preparation

1. Mix blueberries, lemon juice in a small pan and cook on medium heat until blueberries start to plump up.
2. Blend lemon juice, mint and blueberries until smooth.

3. Let cool for a few minutes.
4. Add 4 tablespoons of gelatin and blend until smooth.
5. Pour into a glass dish and refrigerate for 60 minutes.

GREEN SMOOTHIE WITH BLUEBERRY, KALE, GINGER

- 1/2 a bunch Dino kale or Swiss chard, cut out stalks
- 1/2 inch ginger
- ½ cup blueberries
- 5 cups of water
- Blend for 5 minutes

BLUEBERRY, MINT FIZZY

- ½ cup fresh or frozen blueberries
- 12 oz. sparkling water
- ¼ bunch spearmint leaves, chopped
- Blend for 5 minutes

GINGER, BLUEBERRY SORBET

- 10 oz. frozen berries
- 1/2 inch ginger
- Blend for 5 minutes
- Top with homemade yogurt

KIWI, GINGER, MINT SORBET

- 2 frozen kiwis
- ½ inch ginger
- ¼ bunch spearmint
- Blend for 5 minutes

VANILLA, CINNAMON, BANANA SORBET

- 2 frozen bananas
- ¼ tsp vanilla extract
- ¼ tsp cinnamon
- Blend for 5 minutes
- Top with homemade yogurt

BANANA, STRAWBERRY SORBET

- 1 cup frozen strawberries
- 1 banana
- Blend for 5 minutes
- Top with homemade yogurt

GINGER ORANGE, GRAPEFRUIT SORBET

- 1 cup frozen grapefruit slices
- ½ inch ginger
- 1 cup frozen orange slices
- Blend for 5 minutes

Quick Reference Guide

SHOPPING LIST

WEEK 1

☒ MONDAY

GROUND TURKEY HASH

- ½ pound ground turkey
- 1 Tbsp minced ginger
- 2 large carrots, peeled and diced
- Sea salt
- 2 Tbsp olive oil
- 7 water chestnuts

GREEN SMOOTHIE WITH BLUEBERRY, KALE, GINGER

- 1/2 a bunch Dino kale or Swiss chard
- 1/2 inch ginger
- ½ cup blueberries

GINGER STEAMED HALIBUT AND SAUTEED MUSTARD GREENS

- 1 pound halibut
- 1 inch of sliced ginger
- ¼ bunch cilantro
- Lemon slices
- 2 Tbsp olive or red palm oil
- Sea salt to taste
- One bunch of mustard greens

BLUEBERRY, MINT FIZZY

- ½ cup fresh or frozen blueberries
- 12 oz. sparkling water
- ¼ bunch spearmint leaves, chopped

¤   TUESDAY

CHICKEN LIVER PATE

- 1 pound chicken livers
- 1/2 cup olive oil
- 2 tbsp capers
- 3 tsp fresh thyme
- 2 tsp fresh rosemary
- ¼ cup chicken broth

SEARED MACKEREL WITH A SIDE OF MUSTARD GREENS

- 1 pound mackerel
- 2 Tbsp ginger
- 4 cups mustard greens
- 2 Tbsp olive or red palm oil
- Olive oil spray
- 2 Tbsp fresh cilantro
- Pinch of sea salt

BONE BROTH

- 2 lbs chicken or beef bones (or oxtail)
- 2 bay leaves
- 2 tablespoon apple cider vinegar
- 1 teaspoon sea salt

SLOW COOKED CHICKEN

- 3 Lbs boneless, skinless chicken thighs
- 3 carrots, chopped
- Sea salt to taste
- 2 medium zucchinis chopped
- 1/4 cup olive oil
- 1 TB dried thyme
- 1 TB sage
- 1 1/2 cups chicken broth

¤   WEDNESDAY

JUMBO SHRIMP SAUTEED WITH WATERCRESS

- 1/2 cup chicken stock or broth
- 1/4 cup Red Boat fish sauce
- 5 tablespoons olive oil
- 1 1/4 pounds shelled and deveined jumbo shrimp
- 3 tablespoons minced fresh ginger
- One 6-ounce bunch watercress
- 1 tablespoon fresh lime juice

VEGETABLE BROTH

- 3 quarts of water
- 2 sliced carrots
- 1 cup of cubed daikon
- 1 cup of turnips and rutabaga cut into large cubes
- 2 cups of chopped greens: kale, parsley, collard greens, chard, cilantro
- 4 ½ inch slices of ginger

TURMERIC CHICKEN WITH ZUCCHINI AND BASIL

- 2 grilled chicken breasts
- 3 medium zucchinis, sliced thinly
- ½ bunch of basil leaves
- 2 Tbsp olive oil
- 2 tsp Turmeric
- Olive oil spray
- Sea salt to taste

¤   THURSDAY

BLUEBERRY COCONUT KEFIR WATER

- 1 quart coconut water
- 1 cup blueberries
- 3 Tbsp dairy free water kefir grains

GRILLED CHICKEN WRAPPED IN STEAMED COLLARD GREENS WITH CRUNCHY VEGGIES

- 2 chicken breasts
- 1 Tbsp minced ginger
- 3 large carrots, peeled and diced
- Sea salt
- 2 Tbsp olive oil
- ½ daikon radish
- 1 bunch of collard greens

BONE BROTH

- 2 lbs chicken or beef bones
- 2 bay leaves
- 2 tablespoon apple cider vinegar
- 1 teaspoon sea salt

ROSEMARY AND SEA SALT BAKED LAMB CHOPS ON A BED OF KALE CHIPS WITH ARUGULA AND ENDIVE SALAD

- 1 pound lamb chops
- 2 Tbsp minced fresh rosemary
- 2 teaspoons sea salt
- 4 Tbsp olive oil
- 5 pieces of kale
- Olive oil spray
- 1 head of arugula
- 6 heads of endive
- 1 cucumber, sliced
- 1 Tbsp. balsamic vinegar

¤   FRIDAY

HOMEMADE COCONUT YOGURT

- 1 quart coconut milk
- ¼ tsp probiotic yogurt starter
- Yogurt maker

GRILL PAN PORK CHOPS WITH SAUTÉED YELLOW SQUASH AND ARUGULA SALAD

- 2 Pork Chops
- 5 small yellow squash sliced
- ¼ bunch of fresh flat leaf parsley
- 5 Tbsp olive oil divided
- 2 Tbsp balsamic vinegar
- 4 cups arugula
- Sea salt to taste

GINGER, ORANGE, GRAPEFRUIT SORBET

- 1 cup frozen grapefruit slices
- ½ inch ginger
- 1 cup frozen orange slices

BALSAMIC PORK TENDERLOIN ON A BED OF RED KALE

- 1 teaspoon salt
- 1/4 cup balsamic vinegar
- 1/2 cup olive oil
- 1 one pound pork tenderloin
- 6 leaves of Russian red kale

¤   SATURDAY

VEGETABLE BROTH

- 2 sliced carrots
- 1 cup of cubed daikon
- 1 cup of turnips and rutabaga cut into large cubes
- 2 cups of chopped greens: kale, parsley, collard greens, chard, cilantro
- 4 ½ inch slices of ginger

HOMEMADE COCONUT YOGURT

- 1 quart coconut milk
- ¼ tsp probiotic yogurt starter
- Yogurt maker

GINGER CILANTRO TUNA STEAK WITH SAUTÉED SPINACH

- Two 4 oz. tuna steaks (1 inch thick)
- 2 tbsp ginger
- 4 cups spinach
- 2 Tbsp olive oil
- Olive oil spray
- 2 Tbsp fresh cilantro
- Pinch of sea salt

GREEN SMOOTHIE WITH BLUEBERRY, KALE, GINGER

- 1/2 a bunch Dino kale or Swiss chard
- 1/2 inch ginger
- ½ cup blueberries

¤   SUNDAY

GREEN SMOOTHIE WITH BLUEBERRY, KALE, GINGER

- 1/2 a bunch Dino kale or Swiss chard
- 1/2 inch ginger
- ½ cup blueberries

BACON ARUGULA DAIKON AND CARROT SALAD

- 2 strips of bacon
- 1 head of arugula
- 1 small daikon radish, grated
- 1 carrot, grated
- 2 Tbsp olive oil
- 1 tsp sea salt
- 1 Tbsp apple cider vinegar

GRILLED ROSMARY SALMON STEAK WITH STEAMED LACINATO KALE

- 1 bunch Lacinato aka Dino kale
- 1 pound salmon
- 2 sprigs rosemary
- 2 Tbsp olive or red palm oil
- Olive oil spray
- Sea salt to taste

WEEK 2

¤   MONDAY

GRILLED ROSMARY SALMON STEAK WITH STEAMED LACINATO KALE

- 1 bunch Lacinato aka Dino kale
- 1 pound salmon
- 2 sprigs rosemary
- 2 Tbsp olive or red palm oil
- Olive oil spray
- Sea salt to taste

GRILLED CHICKEN BREAST WITH KALAMATA OLIVES AND POWER GREENS SALAD

- 2 chicken breasts
- 20 pitted kalamata olives
- 3 Tbsp olive oil
- Fresh thyme leaves for 3 sprigs
- Olive oil spray
- 2 Tbsp apple cider vinegar
- ¼ bunch ea. of kale, chard, cilantro

JUICY GRASS FED BEEF BURGER WITH CRUNCHY GREEN SALAD

- ½ pound ground beef
- Red leaf lettuce and romaine hearts
- 1 peeled and grated carrot
- 2 Tbsp olive oil
- 2 Tbsp balsamic vinegar
- Sea salt to taste

BONE BROTH

- 4 quarts water
- 2 lbs chicken or beef bones (or oxtail)
- 2 bay leaves
- 2 tablespoon apple cider vinegar
- 1 teaspoon sea salt

BACON WRAPPED CHICKEN THIGHS

- 4 pieces of boneless, skinless chicken thighs
- 4 pieces of bacon
- 3 Tbsp olive oil
- 1 tsp sea salt

⌑ TUESDAY

PAN SEARED YELLOWTAIL WITH SAUTEED SPINACH

- 1 pound yellow tail
- 2 Tbsp olive or red palm oil
- 1 bunch of spinach
- 1 Tbsp minced ginger
- Sea salt to taste

BONE BROTH

- 4 quarts water
- 2 lbs chicken or beef bones (or oxtail)
- 2 bay leaves
- 2 tablespoon apple cider vinegar
- 1 teaspoon sea salt

BALSAMIC MARINATED PORK CHOPS

WITH MASHED TURNIPS AND SAUTÉED COLLARDS

- 1 teaspoon sea salt
- 1/4 cup balsamic vinegar
- 6 Tbsp olive oil divided
- 2 bone in one pork chops
- 1 bunch of collard greens
- 4 turnips
- Sea salt to taste

⌑ WEDNESDAY

LEMON ORANGE GELATINO

- 1 orange
- 1 lemon
- 4 Tbsp unflavored gelatin

RAW ZUCCHINI NOODLES WITH SEASONED GROUND PORK

- 2 large zucchinis, julienned
- ½ pound ground pork
- ¼ bunch chopped fresh basil
- ¼ bunch chopped fresh oregano
- Sea salt to taste
- 3 Tbsp olive oil

VEGETABLE BROTH

- 3 quarts of water
- 2 sliced carrots
- 1 cup of cubed daikon
- 1 cup of turnips and rutabaga cut into large cubes
- 2 cups of chopped greens: kale, parsley, collard greens, chard, cilantro
- 4 ½ inch slices of ginger

TURMERIC CHICKEN WITH ZUCCHINI AND BASIL

- 2 grilled chicken breasts
- 3 medium zucchinis
- ½ bunch of basil leaves
- 2 Tbsp olive oil
- 2 tsp turmeric
- Olive oil spray
- Sea salt to taste

¤   THURSDAY

BACON ARUGULA DAIKON AND CARROT SALAD

- 2 strips of bacon, cooked and chopped
- 1 head of arugula
- 1 small daikon radish, grated
- 1 carrot, grated
- 2 Tbsp olive oil
- 1 tsp sea salt
- 1 Tbsp apple cider vinegar

BUTTER AND OAK LEAF SALAD WITH GRILLED ZUCCHINI AND ACV DRESSING

- 1 head of butter leaf lettuce
- 1 head of oak leaf lettuce
- 2 Tbsp apple cider vinegar
- 3 Tbsp olive oil, divided
- Sea salt to taste
- 2 medium zucchinis sliced

BLUEBERRY SPEARMINT GELATINO

- 1 cup blueberries
- 1/2 cup lemon juice
- ¼ bunch spearmint leaves
- 4 Tbsp unflavored gelatin

GRILLED TRI-TIP WITH ARUGULA SALAD

- 4 cups fresh arugula
- 1 carrot peeled and grated
- 2 Tbsp olive oil
- 2 Tbsp balsamic vinegar
- Sea salt to taste
- ½ pound tri-tip steak

¤   FRIDAY

HOMEMADE COCONUT YOGURT

- 1 quart coconut milk
- ¼ tsp probiotic yogurt starter
- Yogurt maker

BANANA, STRAWBERRY SORBET

- 1 cup frozen strawberries
- 1 banana
- Blend for 5 minutes
- Top with homemade yogurt

BONE BROTH

- 4 quarts water
- 2 lbs chicken or beef bones (or oxtail)
- 2 bay leaves
- 2 tablespoon apple cider vinegar
- 1 teaspoon sea salt

STEAMED ALASKAN KING CRAB WITH SAUTÉED BOK CHOY

- Alaskan king crab claws
- One bunch of bok choy
- ½ bunch of cilantro chopped
- 6 Tbsp red palm oil, divided
- Sea salt to taste

¤   SATURDAY

GROUND TURKEY HASH

- ½ pound ground turkey
- 1 Tbsp minced ginger
- 2 large carrots, peeled and diced
- Sea salt
- 2 Tbsp olive oil
- 7 water chestnuts

GRILLED CHICKEN WRAPPED IN STEAMED COLLARD GREENS WITH CRUNCHY VEGGIES

- 2 chicken breasts
- 1 Tbsp minced ginger
- 3 large carrots, peeled and diced
- Sea salt
- 2 Tbsp olive oil
- ½ daikon radish, peeled and diced
- 1 bunch of collard greens

SQUASH PASTA WITH TURKEY, BACON, AND GREENS

- One medium spaghetti squash
- 2 heads spinach

- 2 strips of bacon
- 5 Tbsp olive oil, divided
- ½ pound ground turkey meat
- 1 tsp dried oregano
- 1 tsp dried basil
- Sea salt to taste

⚮ SUNDAY

HOMEMADE COCONUT YOGURT

- 1 quart coconut milk
- ¼ tsp probiotic yogurt starter
- Yogurt maker

DINO KALE AND ORANGE SALAD

- 1/2 head of kale
- 1 orange, wedges cut in thirds
- 2 Tbsp olive oil
- 1 tsp sea salt
- 1 Tbsp apple cider vinegar

JUICY PORTERHOUSE STEAK WITH RUSSIAN KALE

- One 1 pound porterhouse steak
- 4 cups Russian red kale
- 4 Tbsp olive oil
- Olive oil spray
- Sea salt to taste

BLUEBERRY, MINT FIZZY

- ½ cup fresh or frozen blueberries
- 12 oz. sparkling water
- ¼ bunch spearmint leaves, chopped

WEEK 3

¤   MONDAY

HOMEMADE COCONUT YOGURT

- 1 quart coconut milk
- ¼ tsp probiotic yogurt starter
- Yogurt maker

BUTTER AND OAK LEAF SALAD WITH GRILLED ZUCCHINI AND ACV DRESSING

- 1 head of butter leaf lettuce
- 1 head of oak leaf lettuce
- 2 Tbsp apple cider vinegar
- 3 Tbsp olive oil
- Sea salt to taste
- 2 medium zucchinis

BACON WRAPPED CHICKEN THIGHS

- 4 pieces of boneless, skinless chicken thighs
- 4 pieces of bacon
- 3 Tbsp olive oil
- 1 tsp sea salt

¤   TUESDAY

LEMON ORANGE GELATINO

- Juice from 1 orange
- 1 tsp lemon zest
- 1 tsp grated orange zest
- 1 cup boiling water
- 4 Tbsp unflavored gelatin

GINGER STEAMED HALIBUT AND SAUTEED MUSTARD GREENS

- 1 pound halibut
- 1 inch of sliced ginger
- ¼ bunch cilantro

- Lemon slices
- 2 Tbsp olive or red palm oil
- Sea salt to taste
- One bunch of mustard greens

BONE BROTH

- 4 quarts water
- 2 lbs chicken or beef bones (or oxtail)
- 2 bay leaves
- 2 tablespoon apple cider vinegar
- 1 teaspoon sea salt

PAN SEARED YELLOWTAIL WITH SAUTEED SPINACH

- 1 pound yellow tail
- 2 Tbsp olive or red palm oil
- 1 bunch of spinach
- 1 Tbsp minced ginger
- Sea salt to taste

¤   WEDNESDAY

TURMERIC CHICKEN WITH ZUCCHINI AND BASIL

- 2 grilled chicken breasts
- 3 medium zucchinis
- ½ bunch of basil leaves
- 2 Tbsp olive oil
- 2 tsp turmeric
- Olive oil spray
- Sea salt to taste

BONE BROTH

- 2 lbs chicken or beef bones (or oxtail)
- 2 bay leaves
- 2 tablespoon apple cider vinegar
- 1 teaspoon sea salt

BLUEBERRY SPEARMINT GELATINO

- 1 cup blueberries
- 1/2 cup lemon juice
- ¼ bunch spearmint leaves
- 4 Tbsp unflavored gelatin

GINGER CILANTRO TUNA STEAK WITH SAUTÉED SPINACH

- Two 4 oz. tuna steaks (1 inch thick)
- 2 tbsp ginger
- 4 cups spinach
- 2 Tbsp olive oil
- Olive oil spray
- 2 Tbsp fresh cilantro
- Pinch of sea salt

¤   THURSDAY

BLUEBERRY COCONUT KEFIR WATER

- 1 quart coconut water
- 1 cup blueberries
- 3 Tbsp dairy free water kefir grains

GRILLED ROSMARY SALMON STEAK WITH STEAMED LACINATO KALE

- 1 bunch Lacinato aka Dino kale
- 1 pound salmon
- 2 sprigs rosemary
- 2 Tbsp olive or red palm oil
- Olive oil spray
- Sea salt to taste

BONE BROTH

- 4 quarts water
- 2 lbs chicken or beef bones (or oxtail)
- 2 bay leaves
- 2 tablespoon apple cider vinegar
- 1 teaspoon sea salt

RAW ZUCCHINI NOODLES WITH SEASONED GROUND PORK

- 2 large zucchinis
- ½ pound ground pork
- ¼ bunch chopped fresh basil
- ¼ bunch chopped fresh oregano
- Sea salt to taste
- 3 Tbsp olive oil

¤ FRIDAY

HOMEMADE COCONUT YOGURT

- 1 quart coconut milk
- ¼ tsp probiotic yogurt starter
- Yogurt maker

TUNA STEAKS WITH BOK CHOY

- 1 bunch bok choy
- 1 pound tuna steaks
- 2 Tbsp olive or red palm oil
- Sea salt to taste

¤ SATURDAY

LEMON COCONUT KEFIR WATER

- 1 quart coconut water
- ½ cup whole lemon
- 3 Tbsp dairy free water kefir grains

HOMEMADE COCONUT YOGURT

- 1 quart coconut milk
- ¼ tsp probiotic yogurt starter
- Yogurt maker

SQUASH PASTA WITH TURKEY, BACON, AND GREENS

- One medium spaghetti squash
- 4 cups packed spinach
- 2 strips of bacon

- 5 Tbsp olive oil, divided
- ½ pound ground turkey meat
- 1 tsp dried oregano
- 1 tsp dried basil
- Sea salt to taste

⌘   SUNDAY

CHICKEN LIVER PATE

- 1 pound chicken livers
- 1/2 cup olive oil
- 2 tbsp capers
- 3 tsp fresh thyme
- 2 tsp fresh rosemary
- ¼ cup chicken broth or water
- Sea salt to taste

BACON WRAPPED CHICKEN THIGHS

- 4 pieces of boneless, skinless chicken thighs
- 4 pieces of bacon
- 3 Tbsp olive oil
- 1 tsp sea salt

CUCUMBER NORI SALAD

- 2 Nori sheets
- 1 cucumber
- 2 Tbsp apple cider vinegar
- 1 small ginger root
- 1 lime
- 1 carrot
- 1 Tbsp olive oil
- Sea salt to taste

JUICY GRASS FED BEEF BURGER WITH CRUNCHY GREEN SALAD

- ½ pound ground beef
- Red leaf lettuce and romaine hearts
- 1 peeled and grated carrot

- 2 Tbsp olive oil
- 2 Tbsp balsamic vinegar
- Sea salt to taste

WEEK 4

¤ MONDAY

GREEN SMOOTHIE WITH BLUEBERRY, KALE, GINGER

- 1/2 a bunch Dino kale or Swiss chard
- 1/2 inch ginger
- ½ cup blueberries

CARROT GINGER SOUP WITH BACON ON TOP

- 3 Tbsp olive oil
- 7 large carrots, peeled and sliced thin
- Sea salt
- 1 teaspoon minced ginger
- 2 cups or vegetable or chicken stock
- 2 cups water
- 3 large strips of zest from an orange
- Chopped parsley, dill and bacon for garnish

NEW YORK STEAK AND SPINACH SALAD

- 1 pound New York Steak
- 1 head of washed spinach
- 1 carrot peeled and grated
- ½ peeled and sliced cucumber
- 2 Tbsp olive oil
- 2 Tbsp balsamic vinegar
- Sea salt to taste
- Olive oil spray

GROUND TURKEY HASH

- ½ pound ground turkey
- 1 Tbsp minced ginger
- 2 large carrots
- Sea salt
- 2 Tbsp olive oil
- 7 water chestnuts

SKIRT STEAK WITH SAUTEED GREENS

- 1 bunch of chard, chopped
- 1 pound of skirt steak
- 4 Tbsp olive oil
- Sea salt to taste

BONE BROTH

- 4 quarts water
- 2 lbs chicken or beef bones (or oxtail)
- 2 bay leaves
- 2 tablespoon apple cider vinegar
- 1 teaspoon sea salt

OREGANO RUBBED GAME HENS WITH STEAMED RUSSIAN RED KALE AND OAK LEAF SALAD

- 2 Cornish Hens (approx 1 lb. each)
- 1 Tbsp olive oil
- Sea salt
- 3/4 bunch of fresh oregano
- ¼ bunch oregano set aside for cavity
- 1 bunch Russian red kale
- ½ pound of Oak Leak salad
- 4 sprigs of rosemary

⊭   WEDNESDAY

VANILLA COCONUT JELLO-GURT

- 1 quart coconut milk
- ¼ tsp probiotic yogurt starter
- 1 packet of unflavored gelatin
- Yogurt maker
- ¼ tsp vanilla extract

GRILLED CHICKEN BREAST WITH KALAMATA OLIVES AND POWER GREENS SALAD

- 2 chicken breasts
- 20 pitted kalamata olives
- 3 Tbsp olive oil
- Fresh thyme leaves for 3 sprigs
- Olive oil spray
- 2 Tbsp apple cider vinegar
- ¼ bunch ea. of kale, chard, cilantro

VEGETABLE BROTH

- 3 quarts of water
- 2 sliced carrots
- 1 cup of cubed daikon
- 1 turnips and 1 rutabaga
- 2 cups of chopped greens: kale, parsley, collard greens, chard, cilantro
- 4 ½ inch slices of ginger

BLOOD ORANGE CLAY POT CHICKEN

- One 3 pound chicken
- Juice of 1 lemon
- 1 blood orange, cut in half
- 3 Tbsp olive oil
- 5 sprigs of thyme, leaves pulled and chopped
- 5 sprigs of thyme for inside cavity
- 1 Turnip cubed
- 2 carrots, peeled and cut in quarters

- Sea salt to taste

¤   THURSDAY

TUNA STEAKS WITH BOK CHOY

- 1 bunch bok choy
- 1 pound tuna steaks
- 2 Tbsp olive or red palm oil
- Sea salt to taste

HOMEMADE COCONUT YOGURT

- 1-quart coconut milk
- ¼ tsp probiotic yogurt starter
- Yogurt maker

PETRALE SOLE WITH LEMON, OLIVE OIL, THYME AND KALAMATA OLIVES

- 1 1/2 pounds fresh Petrale sole fillets
- 20 kalamata olive, pitted, chopped
- 2 Tbsp olive oil
- Fresh thyme leaves
- Lemon wedges

CHICKEN LIVER PATE

- 1 pound chicken livers
- 1/2 cup olive oil
- 2 tbsp capers
- 3 tsp fresh thyme
- 2 tsp fresh rosemary
- ¼ cup chicken broth or water
- Sea salt to taste

BALSAMIC MARINATED PORK CHOPS WITH MASHED TURNIPS AND SAUTÉED COLLARDS

- 1 teaspoon sea salt
- 1/4 cup balsamic vinegar
- 6 Tbsp olive oil divided

- 2 bone in one pork chops
- 1 bunch of collard greens
- 4 turnip, boiled until soft
- Sea salt to taste

¤ FRIDAY

CINNAMON COCONUT JELLO-GURT

- 1 quart coconut milk
- ¼ tsp probiotic yogurt starter
- 1 packet of unflavored gelatin
- Yogurt maker
- 1/2 tsp cinnamon

BEEF LIVER PATE WITH BACON

- 3/4 pound beef liver
- 1/3 cup olive oil, more to taste
- 2 Tbsp capers
- 3 tsp fresh thyme
- 2 tsp fresh rosemary
- 3 strips of bacon
- 1 Tbsp lemon juice
- Sea salt to taste

GRILLED AHI TUNA WITH GINGERAND SAUTÉED RED CHARD

- 1 one pound Ahi tuna steak
- 1 Tbsp minced ginger
- 5 Tbsp olive or red palm oil
- 1 bunch red chard, chopped

BLUEBERRY SPEARMINT GELATINO

- 1 cup blueberries
- 1/2 cup lemon juice
- ¼ bunch spearmint leaves
- 4 Tbsp unflavored gelatin

PASTURED TRI-TIP, JUMBO SHRIMP AND COLLARD GREENS

- 1 pound tri-tip steak
- ½ pound pre-cooked shrimp
- 1 bunch of collard greens
- 5 Tbsp olive oil
- Sea salt to taste

☐   **SATURDAY**

VEGETABLE BROTH

- 3 quarts of water
- 2 sliced carrots
- 1 cup of cubed daikon
- 1 turnip and 1 rutabaga
- 2 cups of chopped greens: kale, parsley, collard greens, chard, cilantro
- 4 ½ inch slices of ginger

JUMBO SHRIMP SAUTEED WITH WATERCRESS

- 1/2 cup chicken stock or broth
- 1/4 cup Red Boat fish sauce
- 5 tablespoons olive oil
- 1 1/4 pounds shelled and deveined jumbo shrimp
- 3 tablespoons minced fresh ginger
- One 6-ounce bunch watercress
- 1 tablespoon fresh lime juice

HOMEMADE COCONUT YOGURT

- 1-quart coconut milk
- ¼ tsp probiotic yogurt starter
- Yogurt maker

STEAMED ALASKAN KING CRAB WITH SAUTÉED BOK CHOY

- Alaskan king crab claws
- One bunch of bok choy
- ½ bunch of cilantro
- 6 Tbsp red palm oil

- Sea salt to taste

GREEN SMOOTHIE WITH BLUEBERRY, KALE, GINGER

- 1/2 a bunch Dino kale or Swiss chard
- 1/2 inch ginger
- ½ cup blueberries
- 5 cups of water
- Blend for 5 minutes

⌑   SUNDAY

BONE BROTH

- 4 quarts water
- 2 lbs chicken or beef bones (or oxtail)
- 2 bay leaves
- 2 tablespoon apple cider vinegar
- 1 teaspoon sea salt

GINGER ORANGE, GRAPEFRUIT SORBET

- 1 grapefruit
- ½ inch ginger
- 2 oranges

JUICY GRASS FED BEEF BURGER WITH CRUNCHY GREEN SALAD

- ½ pound ground beef
- 1 head of red leaf lettuce and 1 romaine heart
- 1 peeled and grated carrot
- 2 Tbsp olive oil
- 2 Tbsp balsamic vinegar
- Sea salt to taste

SKIRT STEAK WITH SAUTEED GREENS

- 1 bunch of red chard, chopped
- 1 pound of skirt steak
- 4 Tbsp olive oil, divided
- Sea salt to taste

About the Author

Anne Angelone, Licensed Acupuncturist

Bachelor of Science, Cornell University

Master of Science, American College of Traditional Chinese Medicine

Member of Primal Docs The Paleo Physician's Network

And Dr. Kharrazian's Thyroid Docs

✦ Background ✦

My own experience with Ankylosing Spondylitis led me to study the underlying mechanisms of disease expression. After years of investigating and treating leaky gut and autoimmune disease, I have relied on the advanced autoimmune protocol and Functional Medicine to heal these conditions. I personally do well with a low FODMAP plan and love to cook this way. My hope is to share this information with those who would like to treat the underlying causes of "chronic symptoms" and experience greater health sooner than later.

For more info contact: www.paleobreakthrough.com

AUTOIMMUNE RESOURCES:

Sarah Ballantyne, Ph.D. aka: thepaleomom.com

Dr. Datis Kharrazian, Thyroid and Brain Books

Autoimmune and You

Autoimmune-Paleo Cookbook

Practical Paleo by Diane Sanfilippo

Chris Kresser's: Personal Paleo Code

ThePaleoPlan.com

The Paleo Parents Pinterest page

Please check out Sarah Ballantyne's, book The Paleo Approach: Reverse Autoimmune Disease and Heal Your Body, which is now available for pre-order on Amazon.

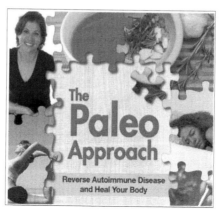

Made in the USA
San Bernardino, CA
14 October 2013